Wellness
The Ultimate Aim

WELLNESS: THE ULTIMATE AIM

Copyright © 2025 Rishikesh Upadhyay
WTL International has obtained
publishing rights.

All rights reserved. No part of this publication may be reproduced in any form or by any electronic or mechanical means, including information storage and material systems, except in the case of brief quotations embodied in critical articles or reviews,
without permission in writing from its author and publisher,
WTL International.

Published by
WTL International
930 North Park Drive
P.O. Box 33049
Brampton, Ontario
L6S 6A7 Canada
www.wtlipublishing.com

978-1-927865-05-7

Wellness
The Ultimate Aim

Rishikesh Upadhyay

DISCLAIMER

I have tried to present my knowledge and experiences faced during an entrepreneurial journey. I have also learned from the experiences of successful business personalities.

I regularly practice mindfulness, various yoga poses, and their benefits on various aspects of health and wellness. I also took other people's opinions and tried to include their views.

This handbook should not be used as a substitute for the advice of a competent wellness professional who is authorized to practice.

ENDORSEMENTS

Dr. Nilesh Rana

I am a medical doctor who has practiced in the United States of America for the last 54 years. I have read numerous books published on the topic of wellness, but this book written by Rishikesh Upadhyay is an eye-opener, and one that is particularly brief but comprehensive.

Wellness refers to a state of optimal wellbeing that encompasses physical, mental, emotional, social, intellectual and spiritual aspects of one's personal life. The seven chapters in this book cover all facets of wellness in a concise fashion. The writing in each chapter is well thought out, written simply and conveyed in language that is easy to understand. It will not bore you.

It is essential to put into practice the information given here in one's regular routines of life. The words enclosed will put you on a path of real fulfillment, having achieved a happy, healthy life. Without any reservation, I recommend *Wellness: The Ultimate Aim* to everyone. "An ounce of prevention is worth a pound of cure."

~**Dr. Nilesh Rana, MD**
Gastroenterologist, USA,
Author & Janmabhumi Columnist

Mr. Rajesh Doshi

"Wellness didn't slow me down. It made me stronger, so from my personal experience, I suggest that everyone considers each aspect of wellness as a first priority to achieve success in other areas of life. Wellness gave me the clarity and resilience I needed to not just chase success, but to truly attain and sustain it. The human body is a temple and not a machine, so taking utmost care of ourselves is the best investment. I never get tired on my journey toward developing world-class plastic extrusion and other plastic products. We have been making machines that are approved and utilized by more than 70 countries in the world. My wellness plays a key part in this. May you find the same in your sphere of life."

~Mr. Rajesh Doshi
*Founder and Chairman, Rajoo Engineers Ltd. &
Rajkot Holistic Health Caretaker,
Holistic Healing Center, Rajkot, Gujarat, India*

Dr. G. L. Jani

Wellness is more than the absence of disease—it is a proactive, holistic approach to health. It emphasizes lifestyle choices, balanced nutrition, quality sleep, stress management, mindfulness, and physical activity—all proven to reduce the long-term risk of chronic illnesses.

For marginalized or underserved populations, wellness practices can offer vital, supplementary pathways to better health. In my practice, I always begin with a thorough understanding of each individual: their symptoms, medical background, lifestyle habits, family history, allergies, and current medications. This comprehensive view allows for tailored guidance—not just to treat illness, but to prevent it, manage it, and promote lasting wellbeing. After decades of caring for a wide range of patients since 1971, my advice remains consistent: focus on improving your health, preventing disease, and maintaining balance. *Wellness: The Ultimate Aim* explores every aspect of wellness, offering practical insights and programs for individuals of all ages.

~Dr. G. L. Jani, MBBS
*Life Member of Gujarat Medical Association,
Pioneer Member of Laughing Club in Una
Treated economically challenged strata of society
for more than 20 years
Una – Rajkot, Gujarat, India*

Mr. Bhargav Joshi

As a reader of *Wellness: The Ultimate Aim*, I have gained a deep and eye-opening understanding of what true wellness means. Before reading the book, I believed that physical health was the only kind of health. Although I've followed a spiritual path and have been involved with spiritual groups in the United States, I never realized that wellness encompasses so many dimensions—mental, emotional, lifestyle, diet, stress-related, and more. This book has inspired me to explore areas of wellness that I had previously overlooked.

As an entrepreneur, I understand firsthand the intense stress that comes with the role—often more than in many other professions. That's why I constantly seek new knowledge and try to apply it to my daily life.

Wellness: The Ultimate Aim has not only broadened my perspective but also given me practical tools to live more mindfully and healthily.

~**Mr. Bhargav Joshi**
*IT Entrepreneur & Governmental Worker,
Maryland, USA*

Dr. V. B. Patel

I have known Rishikesh for over 30 years. We studied together at Lukhdhirji Engineering College in Morbi, where our friendship began. While he pursued a career in India's industrial sector and I followed a path in academia, we have consistently stayed connected, sharing knowledge and experiences over the years.

Rishikesh has always been a person who brings sincerity and dedication to every task he undertakes. He thrives on challenges and demonstrates unwavering commitment in completing even the most difficult assignments. His transition into the field of literature comes as a surprise, yet I have no doubt about his potential to make a meaningful impact here as well.

Having read all his previous books, I admire his approach to learning—he believes in fully absorbing lessons from the past and applying them to the present. Rishikesh's recent work reflects a deep and holistic understanding of wellness, encompassing physical, social, emotional, environmental, spiritual, mental, and financial dimensions. He also explores various wellness programs and emphasizes their importance in our lives.

I sincerely hope his vision reaches a wider audience and contributes positively to society. I am confident that his work will inspire many and help guide them toward a more balanced and fulfilling life.

~Dr. V. B. Patel
Professor & Department Head, Mechanical Engineering Department, LD College of Engineering, Ahmedabad, Gujarat, India

Mr. Vinodbhai D. Trivedi

Wellness encompasses inner peace and pleasure. One can have the same by taking care of mind, body and soul, as we are each made up of all three units. The mind is happy when we think and act positively; the body is happy and strong when we have overall healthy lifestyles; and the soul is happy when we help others, particularly, those who are needy among us. This is because though the body is a highly complex chemical factory, surprisingly, its control valves are emotional, so once you follow the route to total wellness, life will be long, healthy, happy and highly successful. Truly, life will be truly meaningful. One should master the Art of Attach & Detach which truly leads to wellness and away from various evils such as greed, anger, pride, delusion, unrighteousness, ignorance, etc., and will find along with wellness inner peace and pleasure. Hari Om, Hare Krishna...

~Mr. Vinodbhai D. Trivedi
Chairman, Progressive Group (Developers and Builders), Mumbai, Maharashtra, India

Dr. Haresh Dave

As a 40-year practitioner of Ayurveda, I can say that this book is based on the ancient principles of Ayurveda, which identify three fundamental bio-energies—Vata, Pitta, and Kapha—as the governing forces of both physiology and psychology. Each individual has a unique constitution formed by the balance or imbalance of these energies.

When these energies are in harmony, and the digestive system functions properly, it is said that the body attains equilibrium. In such a state, a healthy soul resides within a healthy body, which forms the foundation of good character and a fulfilling life.

This book supports Ayurvedic principles and presents them in a simple, accessible manner. It explores various types of wellness and emphasizes their importance in everyday life.

Ayurveda places great importance on food and its impact on the digestive system. The rise of lifestyle diseases and the modern fast-food culture are considered major contributors to today's critical health issues. This book also offers guidance on healthy eating patterns in alignment with Ayurvedic wisdom.

I firmly believe that true success in life begins with good health. Ayurveda teaches us to maintain wellness not only in the body but in every aspect of life—physical, mental, and spiritual. Find this path as you holistically explore the ultimate aim.

~Dr. Haresh Dave
Ayurvedic Practitioner (of various Ayurvedic camps), Gujarat, India

ACKNOWLEDGEMENTS

First and foremost, praises and thanks to God, the Almighty, for his showers of blessings throughout my work.

On this occasion, I am grateful for all my Vipassana teachers and their guidance.

I would like to express my gratitude to **Mr. Pavan Bhatt** for extending help with respect to editing the content.

I also extend my gratitude to **Dr. Palak Bhatt, Cancer Specialist,** for providing guidance and support during the process. My sincere gratitude towards each health professional who helped me in giving structure to my thoughts. I am grateful for their valuable advice, constructive feedback, and positive appreciation throughout the journey.

I sincerely thank my wife **Mrs. Manisha** and Children **Miss Jalak** and **Master Dev** for their valuable suggestions.

I must express thanks to my brother **Mr. Chintan** for helping to bring my dream to reality by coordinating with the Publisher.

Lastly, my heartfelt regards go to my father for his unconditional love and moral support.

DEDICATIONS

I dedicate this book to all wellness experts and teachers of various mindfulness techniques. I learned so much from psychiatry and mental wellness gurus. They provided me valuable insights while writing this book.

I also learned many things from my father—**Mr. Manuprasad Harilal Upadhyay**. He is a civil engineer and has been practicing yoga since my childhood. This inspired me to present this ancient wisdom. I must thank him for his untiring guidance and support through all kinds of ups and downs throughout my life journey.

TABLE OF CONTENTS

Introduction ...1

Physical Wellness ...7

Social Wellness...21

Spiritual Wellness ...33

Emotional Wellness ...45

Environmental Wellness...59

Mental Wellness ...69

Financial Wellness...81

Conclusion ...91

About the Author ...92

INTRODUCTION

Physical Wellness
- Choices to avoid harmful habits
- Practice behaviours to support body, health and safety
- Intake proper nutritious food
- Follow necessary sleep

Social Wellness
- Building and Maintaining diversity of supportive relationship
- Dealing effectively with interpersonal conflict
- Keep relation with good friends
- Value family supports

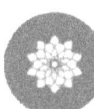
Spiritual Wellness
- Belief and values that provide sense of purpose
- Give meaning and purpose to life
- Behave in alignment with beliefs
- Positive mindset in every situation

Emotional Wellness
- Understanding your own feelings
- Expressing Emotions in a constructive way
- Ability to deal with stress
- Cope with life challenges

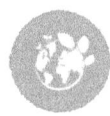
Environmental Wellness
- Organize work schedule
- Keep healthy living area
- Use maximum natural light
- Believe in co-existence of plants and other living things

Mental Wellness
- Pickup New hobbies
- Live as much as possible with nature
- Learn new things
- Give food to the mind such as podcast, research, write anything

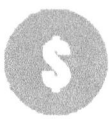
Financial Wellness
- Cash Management
- Loan & Debt Issues
- Budgeting and Saving

INTRODUCTION

What is Wellness?

Wellness is a holistic concept that encompasses various dimensions of health and wellbeing. It is not just physical health. The goal of wellness is to create a balanced and fulfilling life by taking care of each of these areas. Wellness and wellbeing will be used interchangeably throughout this publication. Here are some key aspects of wellness and wellbeing:

Physical Wellness

- **Exercise**: Regular physical activity is crucial for maintaining cardiovascular health, strength, and flexibility.

- **Nutrition**: Eating a balanced, nutrient-rich diet is vital for maintaining energy, supporting immune function, and preventing chronic diseases.

- **Sleep and Preventative Care**: Getting enough restful sleep is essential for recovery, cognitive function, and emotional balance. Regular health check-ups, screenings, and vaccinations help catch issues early.

Social Wellness

- **Healthy relationships**: Building supportive, positive connections with friends, family, and colleagues is important for social health.

- **Community involvement**: Engaging in social or volunteer activities can provide a sense of purpose and connection.
- **Effective communication**: Being able to express yourself clearly and also to listen actively to others greatly enhances relationships and fosters understanding.

Spiritual Wellness

- **Purpose and meaning**: Connecting with a higher purpose or practicing mindfulness can create a deeper sense of fulfillment.
- **Meditation or Prayer**: These practices can offer a sense of peace and help you feel more centered.
- **Values**: Living in alignment with your core beliefs and values contributes to a sense of integrity and peace.

Emotional Wellness

- **Self-Awareness**: Understanding your emotions, triggers, and responses can help manage stress and improve emotional health.
- **Stress Management**: Techniques like deep breathing, mindfulness, and meditation can help reduce stress and improve emotional resilience.

- **Self-Compassion**: Treating yourself with kindness, especially during difficult times, helps maintain emotional balance.

Environmental Wellness

- **Physical Environment**: Creating a clean, safe, and organized space can positively impact your wellbeing.
- **Connection to Nature**: Spending time in nature or bringing natural elements into your living space can enhance emotional and mental health.
- **Sustaining Nature**: Maintaining the planet in a healthy and harmonious state helps secure current and future generations.

Mental Wellness

- **Cognitive Function**: Engaging in activities that challenge the brain, like puzzles, reading, or learning new skills, can improve cognitive health.
- **Mindset**: Cultivating a positive, growth-oriented mindset can foster mental clarity and reduce negative thinking.
- **Emotional Intelligence**: The ability to recognize, understand, and manage your emotions—and empathize with others—plays a huge role in mental wellbeing.

Financial Wellness

- **Financial Wellness** refers to the state of managing your finances in a way that supports your overall wellbeing and peace of mind. It's about having control over your financial situation, understanding how money works in your life, and taking proactive steps to secure your financial future. Like other aspects of wellness, financial wellness isn't just about how much money you have, but how you manage, plan, and prioritize your financial resources.

INTRODUCTION

References

https://www.pureviewhealthcenter.org/the-importance-of-regular-check-ups-preventive-care-at-pureview-health-center

1

PHYSICAL WELLNESS

1.1 What is Physical Wellness?

Physical wellness encompasses the overall health of the body, including fitness, and the ability to carry out daily tasks. It involves adopting strategies that help one to achieve these aims.

1.2 Signs of a Healthy Physical State of Being

Regular Check-Ups

Physical wellness involves regular check-ups. These play a vital role in detecting potential health issues early.

Healthy Body Weight

Maintaining a healthy weight is crucial to reducing the risk of chronic diseases like heart disease, diabetes, and hypertension.

Personal Hygiene

Regular hygiene practices like bathing, brushing teeth, and handwashing help prevent infections and promote general health.

Active Hobbies

Cultivating healthy habits like reducing screen time, spending time outdoors, and nurturing hobbies can enhance both mental and physical wellbeing.

Adequate Sleep

Adequate sleep is essential for physical recovery, mental function, and immune health. Most adults need 7-9 hours of sleep per night.

Stress Management

A healthy handle on stress and the healthy management of anxiety contribute to one's physical health. Chronic stress can weaken the immune system, raise blood pressure, and lead to unhealthy behaviors.

"You can't climb
the ladder of success
with your hands
in your pockets."
Arnold Schwarzenegger

1.3 Benefits of Positive Physical Wellbeing

Physical wellbeing supports long-term bodily health and vitality.

1.4 Elements That Physical Wellbeing Encompasses

Exercise

Aerobic Activities

Walking, running, cycling, swimming, dancing, etc., improve cardiovascular health and endurance. These activities effectively help burn calories.

Strength Training

Resistance exercises such as weightlifting or bodyweight movements (e.g., push-ups and squats) enhance muscle mass, boost metabolism, and strengthen bones.

Flexibility Exercises

Practices like yoga and Pilates improve joint mobility and posture, and they decrease the risk of injury. They also help restore balance. Range of motion exercises help fully engage joints and also contribute to flexibility, mobility and joint function.

Balance Exercises

Stability exercises, such as tai chi, are especially beneficial as we age.

Healthy Eating

Nutrient-Dense Foods

Whole foods like fruits, vegetables, lean proteins, whole grains, and healthy fats provide essential nutrients for energy, immune function, and overall health.

Hydration

Adequate water intake is vital for digestion, nutrient absorption, and maintaining healthy skin.

Moderation

Controlling sugar, salt, and processed food intake decreases the risk of chronic diseases like obesity, diabetes, and heart disease.

Balanced Diet

Macronutrients

The body requires a balance of macronutrients, i.e., carbohydrates, proteins and fats, for energy and bodily functions:

Carbohydrates

Carbohydrates are the primary energy source found in fruits, vegetables, whole grains, and legumes.

Proteins

Proteins are necessary for muscle repair, immune health, and hormone production. Good sources include lean meats, fish, eggs, legumes, tofu, and nuts.

Fats

Healthy fats are important for brain function, cell structure, and hormone production:

Healthy Fats

Monounsaturated (e.g., olive oil, avocado) and polyunsaturated fats (e.g., omega-3s from fish and flaxseeds) support heart health and brain function.

Unhealthy Fats

Trans fats and excess saturated fats (found in fried foods, packaged snacks, and some animal products) can contribute to cholesterol buildup and increase heart disease risk.

Micronutrients

Micronutrients, e.g., vitamins and minerals, also support bodily functions:

Vitamins

Vitamins are important for energy production, immune health, and skin health (e.g., vitamin C, Vitamin D, and the B-vitamins).

Minerals

Minerals are essential for bone health, hydration, and nerve function (e.g., calcium, magnesium, potassium, and iron).

Preventative Healthcare

Elements such as adequate sleep and good hygiene are important elements of physical wellbeing.

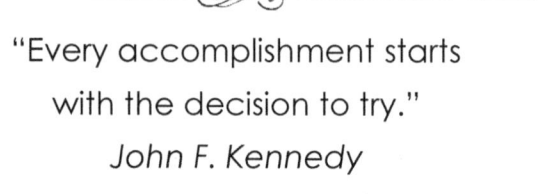

"Every accomplishment starts with the decision to try."
John F. Kennedy

1.5 Special Considerations

Gluten-Free or Dairy-Free

One can seek suitable alternatives like almond milk and gluten-free grains for a better diet.

Special Dietary Needs

Be mindful of your specific nutritional needs, depending on your health, age, activity level, or medical conditions.

Plant-Based Diets

Ensure adequate intake of proteins, vitamin B12, iron, calcium, and omega-3s.

Sports Nutrition

Active individuals may need more protein, carbs, and specific vitamins and minerals for exercise and recovery.

Supplementation (When Needed)

While it's best to get nutrients from eating food, some may require supplements for deficiencies or dietary restrictions. Nutrients like vitamin D, omega-3s, and Vitamin B12 are examples of nutrients that are often supplemented. Consult a healthcare professional before taking supplements, as overuse can be harmful.

1.6 Strategies for Physical Wellbeing

Exercise

Having an Exercise Routine

Incorporate regular exercise into your routine. Balance the activities you engage in to ensure you get enough aerobic exercise, strength training, balance exercises and exercises that will help sustain flexibility.

Healthy Eating

Eating a Variety of Whole Foods

Eat a diverse range of whole foods, including fruits, vegetables, whole grains, lean proteins, and healthy fats, which ensures your body gets all the essential nutrients.

Choosing Nutrient-Dense Foods

Prioritize whole foods like fruits.

Hydration

Ensure an adequate water intake. Water is crucial for digestion, nutrient absorption, temperature regulation, and detoxification. Drinking enough water is often overlooked but crucial for maintaining energy levels and overall health. Aim for at least 8 cups (2 liters) per day, adjusting for activity levels and individual needs. Herbal teas and water-rich foods like fruits and vegetables can also contribute to hydration.

Moderation

Processed and sugary foods often provide empty calories, contributing to health problems like obesity, diabetes, and heart disease. Limit sweets, sugary drinks, and processed snacks, and opt for natural sweetness from fruits. Limit salty and fried foods as well.

Maintaining a Balanced Diet

Make sure your meals include an array of foods that will give you the micronutrients, macronutrients, vitamins and minerals you need.

Fruits and Vegetables

Aim for a colorful variety of fruits and vegetables, as different colors offer distinct nutrients (e.g., green leafy vegetables for iron and folate, orange/yellow fruits for vitamin C and beta-carotene).

Whole Grains

Choose whole grains for sustained energy. Choose whole grains like brown rice over refined grains like white rice for fiber. This supports digestion, blood sugar control, and heart health.

Fats

Focus on unsaturated fats like olive oil, avocado, and fish fat. Avoid excess trans fats and saturated fats by eating less fried foods, packaged foods, and fatty meats.

Portion Control

Eating appropriate portions ensures you get sufficient nutrients without overeating, which can lead to health issues. Tools like smaller plates or portion measurements can help.

Mindful Eating

Focus on the food you're eating—eat slowly, savor each bite, and pay attention to how full you feel to prevent overeating.

Gut Health

Healthy digestion supports overall wellbeing, so include fermented foods like yogurt and sauerkraut in your diet.

Preventative Healthcare

Getting Regular Check-Ups

Schedule physical exams, dental visits, and eye exams regularly. Stay up to date with vaccinations, screenings (cholesterol, blood pressure, cancer), and medical recommendations.

Healthy Body Weight

A balanced diet with healthy eating habits combined with regular physical activity is the most effective way to maintain a healthy weight.

Practicing Good Hygiene

Develop effective hygiene routines. A checklist may help.

Avoiding Unhealthy Habits

Avoid harmful behaviors such as smoking, excessive alcohol consumption, or substance abuse.

Staying Active

Keep a physically active lifestyle by limiting screentime, getting outdoors, and engaging in hobbies that involve movement.

Getting Adequate Sleep

Establishing a regular sleep schedule, managing stress, and creating a calming bedtime routine can improve sleep quality.

Managing Stress

Chronic stress can weaken the immune system, raise blood pressure, and lead to unhealthy behaviors. Practices like meditation, mindfulness, deep breathing, and engaging in relaxing activities can help manage stress.

1.7 Quick Tips

Meal Planning and Prep

Plan meals ahead to make nutritious choices and avoid relying on processed foods. Preparing meals in advance allows for portion control and variety throughout the week.

Eating Meals Regularly

Consistent, balanced meals help maintain energy levels and support metabolism. Skipping meals can lead to overeating later.

Enjoying Food

Focus on savoring the experience of eating, paying attention to textures, flavors, and aromas, rather than using food to cope with emotions or stress.

PHYSICAL WELLNESS

References

https://www.latimes.com/live-well/sleep/story/how-much-sleep

https://www.regencyhcs.com/blog/how-hhas-assist-with-personal-hygiene-and-grooming

https://www.linkedin.com/posts/maalaoui-wassim-38837a216_nutrition-physicaleducation-healthyliving-activity-7350257499226161153-M-fl

https://holisticshealthyguide.com

https://www.nhs.uk/live-well/eat-well/how-to-eat-a-balanced-diet/what-are-processed-foods

https://invisiblecity.uarts.edu/index.jsp/u2D33E/243608/TheArtOfEatingWell.pdf

Takeaway(s) / New Idea(s)

_____
_____
_____
_____
_____
_____
_____

Commitment(s)

_____
_____
_____
_____
_____
_____
_____

Resolution(s)

_____
_____
_____
_____
_____
_____
_____

PHYSICAL WELLNESS

2

SOCIAL WELLNESS

2.1 What is Social Wellness?

Social wellness refers to the ability to create and sustain meaningful, authentic, and respectful relationships with others.

2.2 Signs of a Healthy Social State of Being

Connections

Social wellbeing includes having a supportive network of friends and family. It involves having meaningful, authentic interactions with others.

Boundaries

Establishing healthy boundaries in relationships is key to social wellbeing.

Light Moments

Health includes enjoying social interactions and fun.

Belonging

Social wellbeing includes feeling a sense of belonging.

Diversity

Valuing and embracing diversity are important aspects of social wellbeing.

Communication Skills

Communicating effectively is a sign of positive social wellbeing.

Conflict Resolution

Healthy social wellbeing involves navigating conflicts constructively.

Respect

Demonstrating mutual respect in interactions is a sign of social wellbeing.

Self-Improvement

Improving upon one's social skills is a healthy aspect of one's social wellbeing.

2.3 Benefits of Positive Social Wellbeing

Social wellbeing plays a crucial role in mental and emotional health, helping individuals feel less isolated, more confident, and better equipped to handle stress and anxiety.

Better Mental and Physical Health

Research shows that strong social ties are associated with longer life spans, while loneliness and isolation can harm both mental and physical health.

Emotional Resilience

Social connections help build resilience against emotional challenges, making it easier to cope with difficult situations.

> "Surround yourself with only people who are going to lift you higher."
>
> *Oprah Winfrey*

Assertiveness

A solid social network is an opportunity to foster assertiveness, helping individuals communicate their needs confidently.

Self-Esteem

Positive relationships increase self-esteem, providing emotional support and validation.

Conflict Management

Social wellness encourages the establishment of boundaries and effective communication, which aids in resolving conflicts constructively.

Purpose

A sense of purpose is a benefit of social wellbeing.

Connection

A sense of connection develops from healthy interactions with others.

2.4 Elements That Social Wellbeing Encompasses

Healthy Communication

Being able to communicate clearly, openly and honestly, and listening to others effect social wellbeing.

Healthy Relationships and Staying Connected

Developing and maintaining connections with others contributes to one's social wellbeing.

Community Involvement and Actively Engaging with Others

Structured activities where one engages with the community is a healthy aspect of social wellbeing.

2.5 Special Considerations

How Physical Wellbeing Affects Social Wellbeing

Social wellbeing can be influenced by physical wellbeing. A healthy body often leads to more openness to new experiences and fosters deeper connections with others, contributing to stronger relationships.

Wellness Programs

Wellness Programs in the Workplace

Workplace wellness programs help reduce health-related costs and promote a smoke-free environment.

Wellness Programs in the Community

There are various programs in the community that contribute to wellness. They may be directly or indirectly related to wellness. A book club can increase positive social interactions. A wellness book club can encourage group members to read and discuss topics related to physical, mental, and financial wellness, improving wellness while offering engagement and satisfaction.

School Wellness Programs

Wellness programs in schools promote healthy habits, improve mental and emotional wellbeing, and enhance academic performance. These programs address early physical and mental health concerns while fostering creativity and resilience.

Wellness programs are havens to identify and address early mind/body-related illnesses. Beyond improved academic performance, students also exhibit innovation. A healthy mind and body are achieved leading to the student's holistic growth.

SOCIAL WELLNESS

Wellness programs can benefit both students and staff, and they can have a long-term impact on improving quality of life and educational outcomes.

Wellness programs in schools offer numerous benefits for students, including:

- Encouraging the development of healthy habits
- Teaching time management and stress management skills
- Identifying and addressing health issues early
- Fostering creativity and resilience
- Ensuring holistic growth through physical, mental, and emotional development
- By empowering students with a positive attitude and life skills, schools prepare them for future challenges and success.

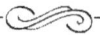

"When we feel love and kindness
toward others,
it not only makes others feel loved
and cared for,
but it helps us also to develop
inner happiness and peace."
The Dalai Lama

Benefits of Specific Types of School Programs

Physical Education

Promotes physical fitness, a key component of overall wellness.

Clubs

Schools can introduce clubs such as dance, yoga, and swimming to encourage activity with others.

Health and Wellness Ambassadors

Teachers can serve as ambassadors to teach students about health promotion and disease prevention.

Counseling Sessions

Counseling can help one manage stress and improve emotional health.

Co-curricular Activities

Help students develop creativity, resilience, and social skills along with others.

Teaching Coping Strategies

Teaching practices like mindfulness can boost productivity and energy in students.

Specific Examples of School Wellness Programs

There are plenty of School Wellness Programs. For example, "School Health & Wellness Program" is a government initiative under the Ayushman Bharat

SOCIAL WELLNESS

Programme aimed at promoting health in schools. "Fuel Up" is a health and wellness program designed for children in schools to foster healthy habits.

2.6 Strategies for Social Wellbeing

Engaging in Healthy Communication

Communicate openly about your feelings. Share your feelings honestly. Express your needs clearly and listen without judgment. Avoid personal attacks and set boundaries. Disagree respectfully and avoid being overly critical. Respect and expect respect from others. When conflicts arise, one should compromise.

Staying Connected

Keep in touch with friends and family regularly. Spend quality time with loved ones to strengthen bonds. Participate in social and physical activities that encourage shared experiences.

Get Involved

Join clubs or organizations to meet new people. Participate in community service or volunteer opportunities. Take classes or attend events at local community centers.

Reaching out to Others

Take the initiative to connect with friends or join a new group.

Reflecting on Your Relationships

Assess whether you are balancing personal time with social interaction and treating others with respect.

2.7 Quick Tips

Focusing on Quality Connections

Instead of accumulating many acquaintances nurture a few deep, meaningful relationships.

Expressing Gratitude

Show appreciation for loved ones through thank-you notes, texts, or small gestures.

Practicing Self-Care

Reflect on yourself: consider how others influence your thoughts and actions; and identify and address your social needs for personal growth. Prioritize your wellbeing while being attentive to the needs of others.

References

https://med.und.edu/education-training/wellness/social-wellness.html

https://www.apa.org/news/press/releases/2019/09/relationships-self-esteem

https://mhwcaustin.org/school-wellness-resources

https://qmis.edu.in/enhancing-student-wellbeing-the-role-of-wellness-programs-in-schools

https://www.walkertownacademy.com/importance-of-wellness-programs-in-school

https://pmc.ncbi.nlm.nih.gov/articles/PMC11673117

https://www.facebook.com/story.php%3Fstory_fbid%3D1093795959416513%26id%3D100063583571808

https://www.westrivereagle.com/articles/at-the-heart-of-it-holding-ourselves-accountable-words-and-actions-impact-others-how-do-you-wield-your-influence

Takeaway(s) / New Idea(s)
_____
_____
_____
_____
_____
_____
_____

Commitment(s)
_____
_____
_____
_____
_____
_____
_____

Resolution(s)
_____
_____
_____
_____
_____
_____

SOCIAL WELLNESS

3

SPIRITUAL WELLNESS

3.1 What is Spiritual Wellness?

Spiritual wellness involves building a connection with both your inner self and the world around you to discover purpose and meaning in life.

3.2 Signs of a Healthy Spiritual State of Being

Well-Defined Beliefs

The ability to articulate your beliefs is a sign of positive spiritual wellness.

Compassion

Caring for others and the environment is an important part of spiritual wellness.

Addressing Needs Appropriately

Balancing personal needs with those of others is a sign of positive spiritual wellness.

Compassion and Values

Acting with compassion in alignment with your values is a strong sign of spiritual wellness.

3.3 Benefits of Positive Spiritual Wellbeing

Developing a sense of purpose and having a set of values that help guide you are benefits of positive spiritual wellbeing. Understanding your beliefs and values can illuminate what drives you, identify potential barriers, and guide rational, responsible decisions.

3.4 Elements That Spiritual Wellbeing Encompasses

Beliefs

Beliefs are assumptions held as true, often shaped by culture, environment, and experience. They may be rigid and not always rooted in fact. Beliefs influence values and morals, sometimes leading to biases or prejudices.

Values

Values are enduring principles that guide decision-making and motivate behavior. They represent how individuals live out their morals through actions, character, and personality. Common values include concepts like fairness, freedom, justice, and equality. Beliefs can evolve into values when an individual grows deeply committed to them. These can manifest in areas like career aspirations, relationships, happiness, and wealth.

Faith

Faith is the confidence or trust placed in a person, concept, or divine power. In religious contexts, faith refers to belief in God or religious teachings. Expressions like "just have faith, it will work out" often offer comfort in stressful or challenging situations. The phrase "all is well," as popularized in the movie *3 Idiots*, also conveys a deeper spiritual meaning tied to hope and reassurance.

Love

Love is a feeling of deep affection, but it is also an action word. One loves others and self by the things they do for the object of their affection. Love can motivate positive actions.

3.5 Special Considerations

Relationship Between Spirituality and Money

While money is important, overvaluing it or constantly chasing it can lead to negative traits such as greed, selfishness, and dissatisfaction. Wellbeing doesn't solely depend on wealth. Your attitude toward money can influence your sense of purpose and fulfilment and this attitude may be governed by your region, belief or values. Acts like charitable giving, volunteering, or community service contribute positively to both personal wellbeing and the wellbeing of others, showing that generosity and support foster a sense of happiness and connection.

Connection Between Spirituality and Aspects of Other Wellness

Spirituality, a deeply personal experience, plays a crucial role in supporting mental and physical health, contributing to overall wellness. It can help you find purpose, peace, and a sense of connection, improving both your relationship with yourself and others. Here are ways spirituality enhances wellness:

Physical Health

Studies suggest that individuals with spiritual beliefs often have lower blood pressure and other positive health indicators.

Relationships

Spirituality can strengthen your relationship with yourself and foster deeper connections with others.

Connection

It can deepen your sense of connection to something greater than yourself and provide comfort and support through spiritual communities.

Mental Health

Spirituality can assist in managing stress and anxiety, boost self-esteem, enhance self-control, and improve confidence. It also provides a sense of strength and clarity during difficult times.

Sense of Purpose

Spirituality can help you find meaning and direction in life, offering clarity on your life's purpose.

Positive Mindset

According to the positive mental attitude philosophy (PMA), a positive mindset is synonymous with hope, optimism, courage, and kindness. A positive mindset is an optimistic approach to life. It involves expecting favorable outcomes while remaining realistic about challenges. This outlook allows individuals to navigate life's ups and downs with resilience and hope. It also means not giving in to negativity and hopelessness even in difficult situations. Positive mindset pillars are:

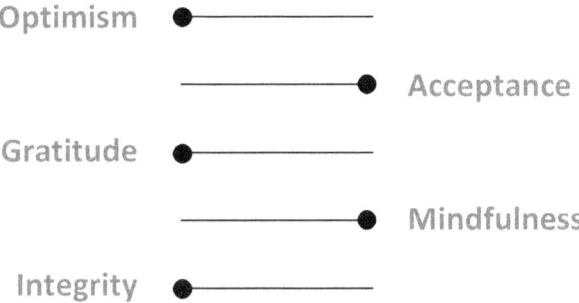

Characteristics of a Positive Mindset

- ✓ Optimism
- ✓ Acceptance
- ✓ Resilience
- ✓ Gratitude
- ✓ Integrity

A positive mindset can have a big impact on your physical and mental health, and can help you succeed in school, work, and other aspects of life.

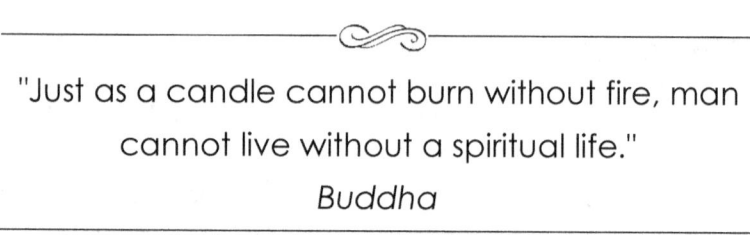

"Just as a candle cannot burn without fire, man cannot live without a spiritual life."

Buddha

3.6 Strategies for Spiritual Wellbeing

Spiritual wellness can be nurtured in various ways including practicing a religious faith, connecting with nature, finding passion in your work, and engaging in meditation. In addition to these are the following:

Prayer and Meditation

To practice spirituality, you might consider activities such as praying, meditating, and engaging in self-reflection and introspection.

Spending Time in Nature

Reconnecting with nature can help purge negative emotions.

Identifying Morals

Define a clear sense of right and wrong.

Making Quiet Time

Find quiet time to recharge.

Declare Your Desires

Speak your intentions into existence.

Reflecting

Reflect on your personal values.

Identifying Your Beliefs

Question and clarify your beliefs.

Evaluating Your Values

Recognize how your values evolve over time.

Tolerance

Understand and respect others' differing values.

Practice mindfulness

Stay present in the moment and observe your thoughts and feelings without judgment.

Embracing a Positive Mindset

Build a positive mindset in the following ways:

Analyzing Life

Starting with a detailed analysis of the world around you can be helpful:

Practicing Gratitude

Take time each day to find things you are thankful for and consider keeping a gratitude journal to reflect on them.

Setting Goals

Establish clear and meaningful goals to provide you with a sense of purpose and accomplishment.

Surrounding Yourself with Positivity

Spend time with uplifting people, listen to music that boosts your mood, and decorate your space with motivating quotes or images.

Practicing Positive Self-Talk

Focus on the good things in your life and trust in your ability to overcome obstacles.

Looking for Opportunities

Emphasize the positive in every situation and be on the lookout for opportunities to grow.

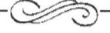

> "You will never be able
> to escape from your heart
> so it is better to listen to
> what it has to say."
> *Paulo Coelho*

3.7 Quick Tips

Enjoying Activities

Activities you enjoy can increase endorphins and make you feel better.

Talking It Out

Talking to close friends or family about what's bothering you can help you feel lighter.

Smiling More

Smiling can change your mood.

References

https://www.thebehavioralscientist.com/list-of-values

https://moonpointer.com/new/2011/09/aal-izz-well

https://hospitalitysearch.co.uk/the-definition-of-a-positive-mental-attitude

https://toolkit.lifeline.org.au/articles/techniques/talk-to-someone-you-trust

https://www.betterup.com/blog/positive-mental-attitude

https://medium.com/%40harshsonwane05/being-positive-in-every-situation-helps-you-grow-a6f698804712

https://geediting.com/9-dire-consequences-of-greed-on-personal-relationships

https://www.facebook.com/groups/peanutscharliebrownlovers.usa/posts/1131195078699699

https://thegrittytherapist.org/the-power-of-resilience-navigating-lifes-challenges-with-strength-and-grace

https://sermoncentral.com/sermons/whatever-rich-o-toole-sermon-on-contentment-283265

Takeaway(s) / New Idea(s)

_____
_____
_____
_____
_____
_____
_____

Commitment(s)

_____
_____
_____
_____
_____
_____
_____

Resolution(s)

_____
_____
_____
_____
_____
_____
_____

SPIRITUAL WELLNESS

4

EMOTIONAL WELLNESS

4.1 What is Emotional Wellness?

Emotional wellbeing refers to the ability to navigate and adjust to life's challenges while cultivating emotions that foster a sense of happiness and fulfilment.

4.2 Signs of a Healthy Emotional State of Being

Sense of Purpose

People with positive emotional wellbeing feel connected to a meaningful purpose and have supportive relationships.

Resilience

With positive emotional wellbeing, a person can quickly bounce back from setbacks and adapt to challenges.

Stress Management

A person with positive emotional wellbeing handles stress effectively and maintains balance.

Self-Kindness

Emotional wellness involves showing compassion towards oneself and positively embracing one's feelings.

Contentment

The emotionally well generally feel satisfied and at peace with their lives.

Self-Esteem

People with positive emotional wellbeing have a positive view of who they are.

Seeking Support

One who knows when to reach out for help from friends or professionals when needed is likely one who exhibits positive emotional wellbeing.

"Your body always speaks—
not in words, but in signals.
Tiredness, cravings, tension—it's not weakness. It's wisdom.
Listen before it starts to scream."

Barbara O'Neill

4.3 Benefits of Positive Emotional Wellbeing

Positive emotional wellbeing is associated with a lower risk of disease, sickness, and injury, faster recovery after being sick or getting injured, improved mental health, stronger relationships and higher self-esteem, as well as better performance at work.

Poor emotional wellness can lead to lower immunity, hypertension, increased illness, relationship issues, trouble concentrating, and difficulties at work.

Emotional wellness can help you avoid going into the fight-or-flight state, which can increase your heart rate, slow down your digestive functions, and make you feel anxious or depressed. Emotional wellness can also help you be more intentional with your communication and make your partner more receptive to what you have to say. In general, one who is emotionally well connects, empathizes, and communicates well with others.

Constructive emotions such as optimism, resilience, and empathy, play a vital role in shaping an individual's development and achievements. For instance, optimism is a powerful mindset that drives motivation and determination.

4.4 Elements That Emotional Wellbeing Encompasses

Stress Management

Emotional wellbeing involves the ability to manage one's stress levels.

Healthy Change

Emotional wellbeing involves the ability to effectively and efficiently adapt to change.

Identifying and Expressing Emotions

Being able to recognize, process, and express a wide range of emotions in healthy ways is important to emotional wellbeing.

Coping with challenges

Emotional wellbeing involves having the skills to deal with uncertainty, stress, and change.

Building relationships

Being able to create positive, satisfying relationships with family, friends, and others is a key area of emotional wellness.

Self-Awareness

Emotional wellness is also knowing your limits, when to press pause, and when to seek support.

Self-Compassion

Being kind to yourself and feeling good about who you are is central to emotional wellbeing.

Conflict Management

Conflict management skills are an important component of emotional wellness. With positive emotional wellness, one typically handles disagreements calmly and constructively.

Decision-Making

One who is emotionally well turns intentions into actions, making informed choices.

Mental Health

Emotional strength is associated with one enjoying higher levels of psychological wellbeing.

Achieving Success

Those who are emotionally well are more likely to reach their personal and career goals.

> "Emotional healing requires more than simply changing how you feel.
> Your emotions are merely symptoms of the problem—not the problem itself,
> even when they hurt."
> *Jessica Moore*

4.5 Special Considerations

Impact of Emotional Reactions

on Varied Areas of Health

A person's overall health is affected by their emotional responses to life's events and one's thoughts. Here are some examples of how emotions impact various areas of health:

Physical Health

When emotional stress activates the fight-or-flight response, this increases one's heart rate and blood pressure. Furthermore, chronic stress can lead to unhealthy behaviors like poor diet, substance abuse, and a lack of exercise.

Mental Health

Negative emotional patterns can lead to anxiety, depression, and PTSD.

Immune Health

Emotional strain weakens immunity, increasing vulnerability to illness.

Anger-Related Illness

Uncontrolled anger can cause severe health issues, including high blood pressure and digestive problems.

Emotional Intelligence (EQ)

EQ, which stands for "Emotional Quotient," is a measure of emotional intelligence. It is described as the ability to recognize, control, and manage emotions effectively in various situations.

Importance of EQ at the Workplace

In the workplace, high EQ is crucial for effective communication. It enables empathy and understanding which help foster collaboration. High EQ also helps workers manage workplace stress and pressures. High EQ individuals make thoughtful, informed decisions. They lead by inspiring others, managing teams effectively, and spotting opportunities. Workplace conflicts are resolved fairly and constructively. People with high EQ can help lessen the stress levels of their coworkers, and people with high EQ tend to be more creative and innovative which boosts company performance.

EQ in Schools

Improved Behavior

Students with high EQ tend to exhibit better behavior and lower stress.

Academic Success

High EQ is associated with better academic performance and higher test scores.

Stronger Relationships

Students with high EQ develop better social connections, which contributes to health, self-esteem and the overall positive experience of school life.

Stress Management

EQ helps students manage stress, contributing to improving grades and overall wellbeing.

Life Success

EQ prepares students for challenges beyond school, fostering personal growth and a balanced life.

Steps Schools Can Take

Schools can help develop EQ in students by implementing social-emotional learning programs and engaging parents in supporting emotional intelligence development.

EQ vs. IQ

IQ (Intelligent Quotient) refers to intellectual abilities, knowledge, and problem-solving skills. It has been said that 99% of the success of the world's greatest leaders is attributable to EQ as opposed to IQ. People with high EQs are consistently found to have better health, quality of life, relationships, and effectiveness.

4.6 Strategies for Emotional Wellbeing

Sleeping

Prioritize adequate sleep in a calm, comfortable environment.

Exercising

Engage in at least 30 minutes of physical activity each day.

Mindfulness

Incorporate mindfulness practices into your daily routine.

Socializing

Participate in group activities that interest you.

Volunteering

Help with causes you care about to gain fulfilment.

Seeking Support

Reach out to mental health professionals when needed. Mental health professionals can provide more specific strategies for personal development.

Other Ways to Improve Emotional Wellbeing

- Managing stress
- Fostering positive social connections
- Being kind to yourself
- Feeling content most of the time
- Feeling you have a strong support network
- Being able to relax
- Feeling good about who you are
- Being self-aware
- Asking for Advice
- Knowing your limits and when to seek support

4.7 Quick Tips

Identifying and Accepting Your Emotions

Take a moment to reflect on what you are feeling and allow yourself to feel those feelings. You can start by asking yourself, "What am I noticing, feeling, or thinking?"

Journaling

Writing helps process emotions and solve problems.

Calming Down

Before you start talking, take a deep breath or use a relaxation technique to calm your mind and body.

Choosing Your Words Carefully

If you're feeling angry, try to calm down before you start talking. You can also try using a word other than "angry" to describe your feelings, like "sad" or "scared."

Starting With "I feel..."

Begin your statements with "I feel," "I felt," or "I have been feeling."

Explaining the Source of Your Feelings

You can start with "My concern is..." to explain the source of your feelings.

Articulating Your Request for Advice

You can say something like, "There's one thing that's off. How could I improve that?" to ask for advice.

Embracing All Feelings

Recognize that all your feelings are okay and important.

Timing

It is not just expressing your feelings, it is finding the right time to express your feelings.

"I Statements"

Use "I" statements Instead of "you" statements.

Employing Technology

You can use an app to help recharge and refocus.

References

https://www.bcbsnd.com/members/health-wellbeing/wellness-articles/rocking-resilience-bouncing-back-from-setbacks-to-catapult-your-success

https://www.cdc.gov/emotional-wellbeing/about/index.html

https://www.nih.gov/health-information/your-healthiest-self-wellness-toolkits/emotional-wellness-toolkit

https://www.nih.gov/health-information/your-healthiest-self-wellness-toolkits/social-wellness-toolkit

https://www.nih.gov/health-information/your-healthiest-self-wellness-toolkits/emotional-wellness-toolkit

https://therapyinanutshell.com/how-to-deal-with-anxiety/

https://www.meetmindful.com/sex-soon-relationship/

https://brainly.in/question/58373852

https://tus.pressbooks.pub/standardsofproficiencysocialcareworker/chapter/chapter-17-lauren-bacon/

https://www.webmd.com/mental-health/mental-health-managing-anger

https://www.helpguide.org/mental-health/wellbeing/emotional-intelligence-eq

Takeaway(s) / New Idea(s)

Commitment(s)

Resolution(s)

EMOTIONAL WELLNESS

5

ENVIRONMENTAL

5.1 What is Environmental Wellness?

Environmental wellness is the practice of living with an external environment that supports personal wellbeing and the health of the planet. It involves being conscious of the impact of one's surroundings on wellbeing, the impact of our actions on the environment, and adopting habits that contribute to sustainability and the preservation of natural resources. This concept encourages individuals to live harmoniously with nature.

5.2 Signs of a Healthy Environmental State of Being

Engaging the Senses With Aspects of the Surrounding Environment

Being aware of one's surroundings and intentionally processing sensory information from the environment is a part of environmental wellbeing.

Design and Cleanliness

Maintaining an environment that suits your personality, is tidy, promotes peace and offers a sense of security can help improve your mood and ability to concentrate. It may also decrease stress.

An Understanding of Sustainability

Being aware of the limits of the earth's natural resources is a part of environmental wellness.

Energy Conservation

Regularly making efforts to conserve energy is part of a healthy environmental wellbeing.

Recycling

Routinely recycling items like paper, cans, plastic bottles, and glass is a healthy practice.

Limiting Pollution

Efforts to avoid polluting the air, water, or Earth as much as possible is a healthy practice for wellbeing.

Living Peaceably With Others

Fostering an environment where one lives in harmony with others is positive environmental wellbeing.

5.3 Benefits of Positive Environmental Wellbeing

The relationship between humans and the environment is fundamental to both personal wellbeing and sustainability. The self-awareness aspect of environmental wellbeing is vital for personal and professional growth, as it enhances decision-making, helps build healthier relationships.

Coexistence

Coexistence encompasses living at the same time and in the same space with other human beings and other life forms without negatively impacting one another. It is fundamental to environmental wellbeing. Some of the benefits of coexistence are:

Social Stability

By reducing conflicts, coexistence helps create more stable societies, fostering peace and understanding.

Common Interests

Coexistence encourages collaboration toward common goals, building a collective future.

Advancing Society

Blending cultures and perspectives leads to the creation of new ideas, enriching societies.

Sustainable Development

Coexistence is crucial for a future where humans live harmoniously with nature, ensuring the planet's resources are available for future generations.

Reaching Agreements

By promoting dialogue and mutual respect, coexistence facilitates solving problems and reaching agreements more effectively.

Empathetic Communities

Coexistence fosters empathy and understanding, leading to more compassionate communities.

---

*"Earth provides enough
to satisfy every man's needs,
but not every man's greed."*
Mahatma Gandhi

5.4 Elements That Environmental Wellbeing Encompasses

Awareness

Awareness refers to the state of being cognizant of our surroundings, thoughts, and actions. There are different types of awareness that contribute to both personal growth and environmental wellness:

Peripheral Awareness

Peripheral awareness is the ability to process information from all five senses at the edges of our attention, such as noticing sounds or movements in the background while focusing on a task.

Sensory Awareness

Sensory awareness is focusing on specific sensory experiences, like noticing textures, smells, or sounds. This practice can help you remain more attuned to the present moment and increase mindfulness. It also helps improve your ability to remain alert to what is happening around you without judgment.

Self-Awareness

The ability to recognize and understand your own thoughts, emotions, and behaviors, and how they affect others is self-awareness. It involves understanding self, your strengths, challenges, and needs. It involves understanding others, the needs and feelings of others and recognizing how your behavior impacts others. It also involves self-assessment, assessing yourself against standards or goals to encourage positive change.

Coexistence

Coexistence is accepting animals or other living things and respecting them and their differences and not using violence against them. In the context of environmental wellness, coexistence also involves the harmonious relationship between humans and nature, as well as between diverse communities. There are a number of values that are necessary for coexistence:

Mutual Respect

Mutual respect is acknowledging and respecting each other's rights, sovereignty, and differences.

Non-Aggression

Non-aggression is a commitment to peaceful relations, free of violence or harm.

Non-Interference

Non-interference is respecting each other's internal affairs and autonomy.

Equality

Equality is ensuring equal treatement and fairness for all parties involved in a particular context.

Peaceful Coexistence

Peace thrives when living together peacefully and collaboratively.

Tolerance

Tolerance involves embracing differences and maintaining an open mind.

Dialogue

Dialogue is engaging in open communication to foster understanding and resolve conflicts.

> A nation that destroys its soils
> destroys itself.
> Forests are the lungs of our land,
> purifying the air
> and giving fresh strength
> to our people.
> Franklin D. Roosevelt

5.5 Strategies for Environmental Wellbeing

Observe the Natural Environment

While strolling in a natural setting, make the effort to consciously notice your surroundings. Engage your eyes, ears, and nose, and note the overall ambience.

Sensory Opportunities

Sensory skills can be nurtured by providing opportunities to explore new sensations, especially for children.

Practicing Introspection

Practice activities like journaling, self-assessment challenges, and reflecting on personal values to help foster self-awareness.

Being Aware

Make time to focus on understanding how your actions affect the environment and recognize how the environment impacts your health and wellbeing.

Respecting Nature

Learn to value the interconnectedness between human life and the natural world, ensuring that both are respected and preserved.

Contributing to a Sustainable Lifestyle

Adopt habits that conserve resources, such as energy conservation, recycling, and minimizing waste.

Spending Time in Nature

We, as human beings, must spend time with nature to improve wellbeing and reduce stress. This also fosters a deeper appreciation for the environment.

Advocating for the Natural Environment

Contribute to environmental sustainability and strive for sustainability in decision-making.

Creating Supportive Built Environments

Design your home and workspace to be nurturing and pleasant, contributing to both mental health and environmental sustainability.

Making a Positive Impact

Be mindful of the broader effects of your actions, advocating for fair treatment of all people.

5.7 Quick Tips

Self-Assessment Challenges

For self-assessment challenges, you can explore one specific aspect of your life at a time, like how you spend your money or identify your values.

Journaling

You can express how you feel, your goals, and reflect on your day using a journal.

References

https://www.joinblink.com/intelligence/open-communication-importance

ENVIRONMENTAL WELLNESS

Takeaway(s) / New Idea(s)

_____
_____
_____
_____
_____
_____
_____

Commitment(s)

_____
_____
_____
_____
_____
_____

Resolution(s)

_____
_____
_____
_____
_____
_____

6

MENTAL WELLNESS

6.1 What is Mental Wellness?

Mental wellness refers to a positive state of mental health, where a person can manage daily life, even in challenging times. It is more than the absence of mental illness. Mental health is closely linked with a person's emotional, psychological, and social wellbeing. It influences how we think, feel, and act, and is vital at every stage of life. It is our right and has an important role in our personal development, community life, and socio-economic development. Mental health conditions can vary in severity, encompassing mental disorders, psychosocial disabilities, and other mental states. Mental illness is influenced by biological factors (e.g., genetics or brain chemistry), life experiences (e.g., trauma or abuse), and one's family history of mental health issues. One's living conditions, daily events, social relationships, sleep and eating habits also influence mental wellness.

6.2 Signs of a Healthy Mental State of Being

Stable Mood

Positive mental wellbeing is marked by a stable mood, optimism and positivity.

Social Engagement

Engaging in social activities is a sign of positive mental wellbeing.

Cognitive Function

Being able to concentrate, remember, and think rationally are signs of mental wellbeing.

6.3 Benefits of Positive Mental Wellbeing

Individuals with good mental wellness can realize their potential, feel secure and safe, thrive in everyday activities, manage stress and challenges effectively, work, and contribute to society.

6.4 Elements That Mental Wellbeing Encompasses

Mental health issues encompass a wide range of conditions that affect thoughts, emotions, and behaviors. Common mental health disorders include:

Depression

Depression is linked to early life experiences, some other life experiences, and social stressors.

Bipolar disorder

Bipolar disorder involves mood drastic mood swings.

Schizophrenia

Schizophrenia is a psychotic disorder that causes inaccurate and erratic thinking, emotions, and perceptions of reality. It often involves paranoia, delusions and perceptions of sensory information that is not actually there.

Post-Traumatic Stress Disorder (PTSD)

PTSD results from experiencing or witnessing traumatic events. It leads to fear, anxiety, flashbacks and emotional distress.

Eating Disorders

Eating disorders are disruptions in eating behaviors.

Obsessive-Compulsive Disorder (OCD)

OCD is characterized by repetitive behaviors or thoughts.

Personality Disorders

Personality disorders include disorders like borderline personality disorder, and antisocial personality disorder.

Substance Use Disorders

Substance abuse disorder involves addiction to drugs or alcohol.

Attention-Deficit/Hyperactivity Disorder (ADHD)

ADHD affects concentration, behavior, and learning abilities, particularly intensifying during adolescence.

6.5 Special Considerations

The Difference Between Mental Health and Mental Wellness

While mental health refers to an individual's current emotional, psychological, and social state, mental wellness encompasses a broader, more proactive, and positive view of mental functioning. Mental health is often linked to the absence of distress. Mental wellness is a positive state focused on overall wellbeing.

Symptoms of Mental Health Issues

Symptoms of mental health issues can vary, but common signs include:

Mood Changes

Sudden shifts in emotions or feeling persistently depressed or irritable can be signs of mental illness.

Withdrawal

Avoiding social activities or losing interest in previously enjoyed activities can be signs of mental illness.

Sleep or Appetite Changes

Significant alterations in sleep patterns or appetite can be a sign of mental illness.

Cognitive Issues

Difficulty concentrating, memory problems, or irrational thinking can be signs of mental illness.

Self-Harm

Engaging in behaviors that cause physical harm is a sign of mental illness.

Suicidal Thoughts

Thoughts or statements about self-harm or suicide are a sign of mental illness.

Physical Symptoms

Unexplained physical issues like headaches or back pain can even be signs of mental illness.

Other Symptoms of Mental Illness

Other indicators of mental illness can include feelings of hopelessness, excessive guilt, extreme anger, hallucinations, substance abuse, or changes in sexual behavior. If any of these symptoms are present, it is crucial to consult a healthcare provider or mental health professional.

Mental Health Issues in the Teenage Years

While intense feelings are a normal part of growing up and adolescence, during adolescence, mental illness is often marked by more intense emotional and psychological ups and downs. Many adult mental health disorders begin during childhood or adolescence.

Promoting Mental Wellbeing in Schools

There are several ways to support mental wellbeing in school environments:

Teaching Social and Emotional Skills

Integrating social-emotional learning (SEL) into the curriculum helps students build empathy, self-regulation, and communication skills.

Practicing Mindfulness

Mindfulness techniques can aid stress management and emotional regulation.

Creating a Supportive Environment

Positive classroom climates, including cooperative learning, foster wellbeing.

Improving the Physical Environment

Updating school furniture and creating safe spaces enhances student comfort.

Encouraging Healthy Eating

Providing healthy food options and partnering with parents on nutrition can have a great impact on the mental health of students.

Hosting "Tea & Talk" Sessions

Creating informal spaces for students and staff to share and discuss challenges can also be helpful.

Providing an Anonymous Feedback System

An anonymous postbox for students to express concerns helps teachers address issues.

> "Success is not final, failure is not fatal:
> It is the courage to continue
> that counts."
> Winston Churchill

6.6 Strategies for Mental Wellbeing

Strategies for Diagnosed Mental Illnesses

How to Manage Mental Health Problems

Mental health conditions can be managed through psychotherapy, psychiatric medications, lifestyle changes, and peer or self-help interventions. They are also treatable with a number of other therapies available to assist in managing them. Some therapeutic approaches include expressive therapies, self-compassion, social-emotional learning, meditation, lucid dreaming, and spiritual counselling.

Engaging in Psychotherapy

Often called talk therapy, psychotherapy involves discussing your feelings and condition with a mental health professional. You may use psychotherapy help develop coping mechanisms and manage symptoms. It can be conducted individually, in groups, or with family members.

Taking Medication

Some mental illnesses respond well to medication, such as antidepressants and antipsychotics. These medications alter brain chemistry to reduce symptoms and should be taken as prescribed.

Using Alternative Therapies

For some conditions, alternative therapies like herbal remedies, massages, acupuncture, yoga, or meditation may offer relief.

Brain Stimulation Therapies

When medication does not help, you might use brain stimulation therapies like electroconvulsive therapy (ECT) which may be recommended. ECT involves stimulating the brain with electricity while under anesthesia.

Utilizing Social Supports

Seeking support from family, friends, and peer groups, along with seeking education on managing the condition, is crucial.

Psychiatric Hospitals

In cases of severe mental illness or when there is a risk of self-harm or harm to others, hospitalization may be necessary.

Engaging in Activities That Improve Mental Wellness

Some activities are particularly effective at helping to manage mental illness such as physical exercises, artistic endeavors, volunteering, spending time with loved ones, eating nutritious food, and completing personal goals. Engage in them.

Strategies for Mental Wellbeing in General

Learning Continuously

Learn new things. It strengthens brain connections.

Prioritize Sleep

Make time for sleep and cultivate good sleeping habits. For instance, turn off your devices and put work away close to bedtime.

Exercising and Music

Exercise, especially with music. This boosts cognitive abilities.

Self-Care

Take time to nurture yourself, whether through relaxation, hobbies, or pampering. Self-care is essential for maintaining balance. Make time for yourself a priority

---

"It does not matter
how slowly you go
as long as you
do not stop."
Confucius

MENTAL WELLNESS

6.7 Quick Tips

Experimenting With Different Methods

There is no one-size-fits-all approach to improving mental wellness. Try various methods that might help to determine what works best for you.

Practicing Mindfulness

Be present and aware in the moment. It helps reduce anxiety and increase emotional well-being.

Engaging in Calming Activities

Engage in calming activities like meditation, yoga, or deep relaxation. Ensure you get enough sleep for mental clarity and emotional well-being.

A Sleep Schedule

Have a routine bedtime. A good sleep schedule enhances brain function.

Practicing Gratitude

Regularly reflect on what you're grateful for. This can improve your mood and your outlook on life.

References

https://neurowellnessspa.com/what-causes-mental-illness/

https://www.riseabovetreatment.com/dual-diagnosis-treatment-centers

https://televerohealth.com/when-you-start-avoiding-things-you-used-to-love/

https://navis-health.com/menopause-rage-understanding-and-managing-emotional-turmoil-during-menopause

https://actforyouth.org/adolescence/mental-health/

https://studentreasures.com/blog/social-emotional-learning/social-emotional-learning-benefits-students/

https://thrombosis.org/patients/patient-articles/the-power-of-meditation-and-mindfulness-for-stress-reduction

https:///search?sca_esv=310e4980e99ea993

https://www.newleaders.org/blog/social-emotional-learning-ways-for-school-leaders-to-support-students

MENTAL WELLNESS

Takeaway(s) / New Idea(s)

___

Commitment(s)

___

Resolution(s)

7

FINANCIAL WELLNESS

7.1 What is Financial Wellness?

Financial wellness is a crucial aspect of maintaining personal and organizational wellbeing. It involves the process of managing, controlling, and reporting on financial resources to ensure stability and growth.

7.2 Signs of a Healthy Financial State of Being

Financial Independence

Financial independence, the ability to care for one's needs tied to the costs of one's life and one's family is a sign of positive financial wellness.

Financial Freedom

Financial freedom means having enough resources to live life according to your own terms. It involves being able to live out your goals without hindrances (within reason.) This might mean retiring early, traveling, or simply living without financial stress.

Savings

Having savings for the future and an emergency fund is a sign of financial wellbeing.

Investments

Having investments or investment plans are a sign of financial wellbeing.

Understanding Finances

Understanding money and your particular financial habits are an indication of strong financial wellbeing.

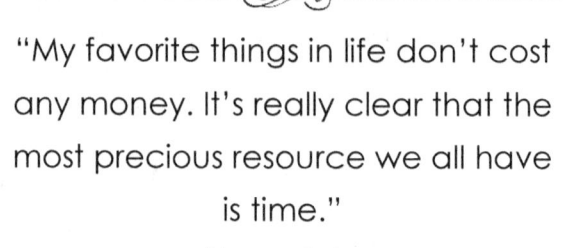

"My favorite things in life don't cost any money. It's really clear that the most precious resource we all have is time."
Steve Jobs

7.3 Benefits of Positive Financial Wellbeing

Achieving financial wellbeing helps you enjoy peace of mind and autonomy over your life choices. Positive financial wellbeing fosters a sense of self-sufficiency which is good for emotional and mental wellbeing. It also greatly contributes to reducing stress surrounding financial strain. Financial wellness helps meet your needs an can support a healthier, more enjoyable, more comfortable lifestyle.

7.4 Elements That Financial Wellbeing Encompasses

Budgeting

A well-structured budget helps track income and expenses, providing clarity on spending patterns. It ensures that resources are allocated effectively for both short-term needs and long-term savings goals. A clear budget aids in making informed financial decisions, prevents unnecessary debt, and allows for planning toward future goals.

Living Within Your Means

Financial wellness requires discipline in managing income and expenditure. This means prioritizing needs over wants and avoiding lifestyle inflation. Living below your means provides an opportunity to save, invest, and build long-term wealth.

Setting Long-Term Goals

Financial independence involves setting clear, actionable goals, such as paying off debt, saving for a down payment on a house, or achieving retirement. These goals give purpose to your financial decisions and guide you toward the life you want.

Financial Literacy

Understanding personal finance is the foundation of financial wellness. It involves knowledge of budgeting, saving, investing, and managing debt. It also includes understanding how to read credit reports, interest rates, and the tax implications of your financial decisions.

Improving Financial Knowledge

Continually learning about personal finance is crucial to making sound financial decisions. This could involve reading books, taking courses, or consulting with financial professionals. Gaining financial knowledge reduces the likelihood of making costly mistakes.

Building an Emergency Fund

An emergency fund acts as a safety net for unforeseen circumstances such as job loss, medical emergencies, or unexpected repairs. Financial experts recommend saving 3-6 months' worth of living expenses to protect yourself from financial stress.

Saving for Future Goals

Planning for goals such as buying a home, funding education, or retirement is essential for long-term financial health. Consistently saving, automating transfers to savings accounts, and setting clear goals make it easier to reach these milestones without feeling overwhelmed.

Understanding and Managing Debt

Debt is a common part of life, but it's important to understand the difference between good and bad debt. High-interest debt (like credit card debt) can quickly spiral out of control, whereas low-interest debts (like mortgages or student loans) are more manageable. Keeping debt in check is critical for maintaining financial wellness.

Debt Repayment Strategies

Common strategies for debt repayment include the debt snowball method (paying off smaller debts first to gain momentum) and the debt avalanche method (focusing on paying off higher-interest debt first). Both strategies can help reduce debt more efficiently.

Saving

Saving is setting aside money that will not be spent immediately. It is intended for short-term needs. Saving is an important aspect of financial wellness.

Investing

Investing is setting aside money for the future. It is aimed at growing wealth over the long term.

Retirement Planning

Retirement planning, such as contributing to 401(k), IRA, or pension plans, ensures financial security in later years. A diversified portfolio of investments—stocks, bonds, real estate, and mutual funds—helps mitigate risk and grow wealth over time.

Building Wealth

whereas saving preserves the value of your assets, investing helps build wealth by earning returns on your money. Understanding various investment options and their risks is essential to making informed decisions and achieving financial goals.

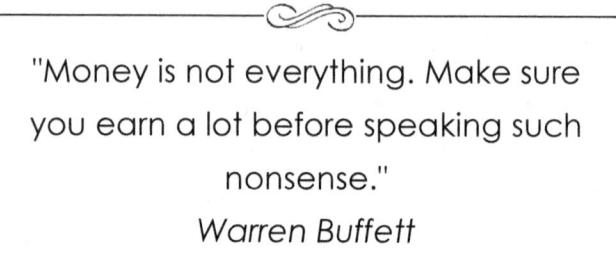

"Money is not everything. Make sure you earn a lot before speaking such nonsense."
Warren Buffett

7.5 Special Considerations

The Connection Between Financial Wellness and Other Wellness

Financial stress can have a direct impact on physical, mental, and emotional health. Money worries can lead to anxiety, poor sleep, or even physical ailments like headaches or high blood pressure. Achieving financial wellness can reduce stress and contribute to better health, while poor financial management can lead to constant worry and affect your overall sense of wellbeing. Having adequate finances can give you more nutritional options, access to facilities such as gyms where you can exercise, the social and community programs, healthcare, medications and nutritional supplements you might need for your physical, social and mental health. By improving your financial wellness, you not only create a more secure financial future, but you also enhance your ability to enjoy life, pursue your goals, and experience a greater sense of freedom in varied aspects of life.

7.6 Strategies for Financial Wellbeing

Tracking Your Spending

Understand where your money goes each month and identify areas where you can cut back. Tracking spending can foster conscious financial decisions.

Creating a Budget

Draft a budget that reflects your income, expenses, and savings goals. Set limits on discretionary spending to help stay within your means.

Saving Consistently

Regular savings, even in small amounts, can add up over time. Setting up automatic transfers makes saving effortless.

Paying Off High-interest Debt

Paying down high-interest debt, such as credit card balances, will free up more money for savings and investments.

Investing Wisely

Start investing early, whether through retirement accounts or personal investment portfolios, to build wealth over time.

Checking Your Credit

Regularly review your credit report for errors, and work on improving your credit score by paying off debts and making on-time payments.

Building Healthy Financial Habits

Financial habits, such as budgeting, saving, and tracking expenses, are vital.

Financial mindfulness

Being mindful of your financial decisions means regularly reviewing your financial situation, adjusting when necessary, and staying proactive in managing your resources.

Emotional Approach to Money

The way you think and feel about money influences your financial habits. A positive, empowered mindset helps in making smart financial decisions, while stress or fear about money can hinder your financial progress. Shifting toward a mindset that focuses on financial empowerment and control can help you improve your financial wellbeing.

7.7 Quick Tips

Focusing

Stay disciplined, informed, and committed to your long-term financial goals.

Practicing Consistency

Just like physical wellness, financial wellness requires consistent attention and maintenance.

References

https://www.investopedia.com/terms/e/emergency_fund.asp

https://www.bmc.net/blog/finance-and-accounting-articles/why-personal-financial-planning-is-important

https://thegildgroup.com/financial-health-metrics/

https://www.usbank.com/financialiq/invest-your-money/investment-strategies/saving-vs-investing-whats-the-difference.html

https://financialwellness.pitt.edu/saving-investing

https://money.pro/blog/2023/09/07/financial-wellness-achieving-balance-and-peace-of-mind

https://www.gobankingrates.com/saving-money/savings-advice/how-much-should-you-save-each-month

FINANCIAL WELLNESS

Takeaway(s) / New Idea(s)

___
___
___
___
___
___
___

Commitment(s)

___
___
___
___
___
___
___

Resolution(s)

___
___
___
___
___
___
___

CONCLUSION

Wellness is a continual process of self-improvement and adaptation, and it requires regular attention across all areas of life. It is about finding balance and making choices that nurture and support your overall wellbeing. Most importantly, wellness is attainable. It involves implementing an achievable set of strategies. Once the components of wellness are identified—those of physical health, social health, spiritual health, emotional health, environmental health, mental health, and financial health—they can be attempted. *Wellness: The Ultimate Aim* is an attempt to identify these components and start you on your path to the richness a truly healthy life bestows.

ABOUT THE AUTHOR

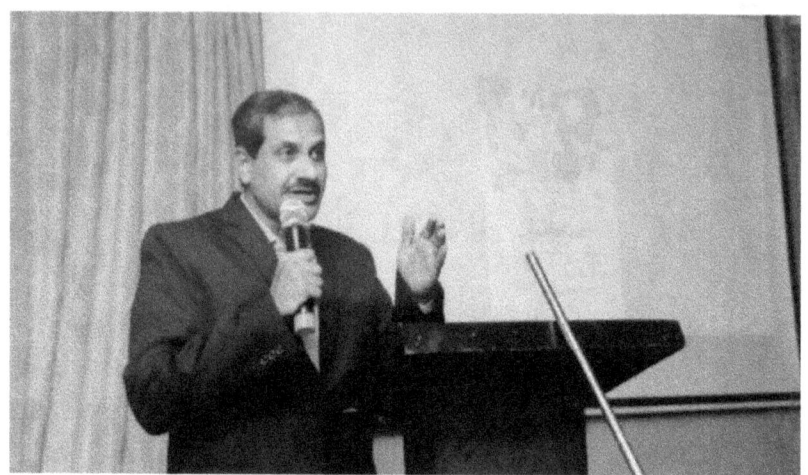

Rishikesh's passion for continuous learning has driven him to expand his knowledge through diverse educational programs. To fulfill his belief for continuous learning, he did short duration courses from **Indian Institute of Management (IIM) Calcutta**, **IIM Bangalore** and **International Business Operation** from Indira Gandhi National Open University (IGNOU) as well as **Post Graduate Diploma in Management (Systems)** from South Indian Education Society (SIES) college of Management Studies, Mumbai.

Rishikesh is a life member of **Institute of Directors** (IoD), **Bombay Management Association** (BMA - Mumbai), **National Human Resources Development Network (NHRDN)**, and the **Indian Society for Training and Development (ISTD)**. He thrives on exploring new perspectives and innovative ideas. His commitment to innovation and doing things differently has always led him to venture into uncharted territories.

As an avid member of Toastmasters International, Rishikesh was awarded the titles of **"Competent Communicator" and "Competent Leader."**

As the **founding secretary** of Progressive's Signature Cooperative Housing Society (CHS) Ltd., Navi Mumbai, Rishikesh played a crucial role in setting up and managing the residential complex, including finalizing service contracts and opening the society bank account. He deeply values India's rich culture, ancient knowledge and great contribution to humanity such as Yoga, Ayurveda and other knowledge, which Western scientists have also supported through their inventions. He is life member of **ISKCON** and practices Yoga taught by **PATANJALI** teachers. He also did various courses of **ART OF LIVING** and regularly practices **VIPASSANA** and its ideals taught by Goenka Guruji. Rishikesh has done shibirs at Igatpuri, Belapur, Global Vipassana Pagoda at Mumbai, Rangpar at Rajkot, and Palitana and Bada in Kutch. The Shibirs take place for durations ranging from between a few hours to 10 days.

Rishikesh has penned 5 unique books: *"The Corporate Yoga Anatomy," "Pearls of Wisdom," "Cycling – The Real Wealth", "Wellness: The Ultimate Aim"* and *"AI V/s. Spirituality."* He has also written few blogs on various subjects.

LinkedIn: https://www.linkedin.com/in/rishikesh-upadhyay-2020/?originalSubdomain=in

www.ingramcontent.com/pod-product-compliance
Lightning Source LLC
Chambersburg PA
CBHW071641080526
44586CB00013BA/1340